ABORTION AND THE BLACK CHURCH

Breaking the Silence

Dr. Barbara C. Crawford

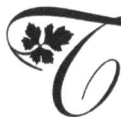

WWW.TRUEVINEPUBLISHING.ORG

Abortion and the Black Church
Dr. Barbara C. Crawford

Published by
True Vine Publishing Co.
810 Dominican Dr.
Nashville, TN 37228
www.TrueVinePublishing.org

Printed in the United States of America—First printing.

DEDICATION

I dedicate this book to my former pastors, all of whom greatly contributed to my spiritual formation and theological development: Rev. Charlie Hoge (deceased), Rev. William Gardner (deceased), and Rev. Percy Clark (deceased), Mt. Calvary Missionary Baptist Church (Herman Street); Rev. Dr. Kenneth Robinson and Rev. Sidney Bryant, Payne Chapel African Methodist Episcopal (AME) Church. To God be the Glory!

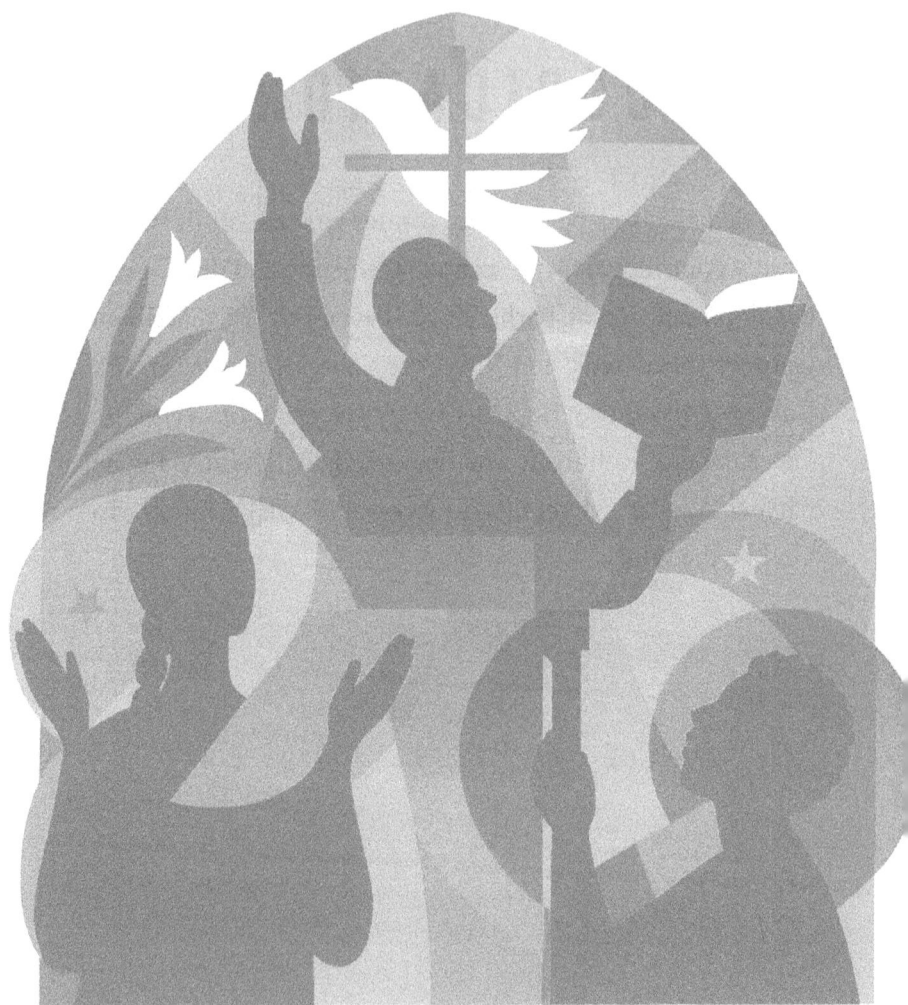

TABLE OF CONTENTS

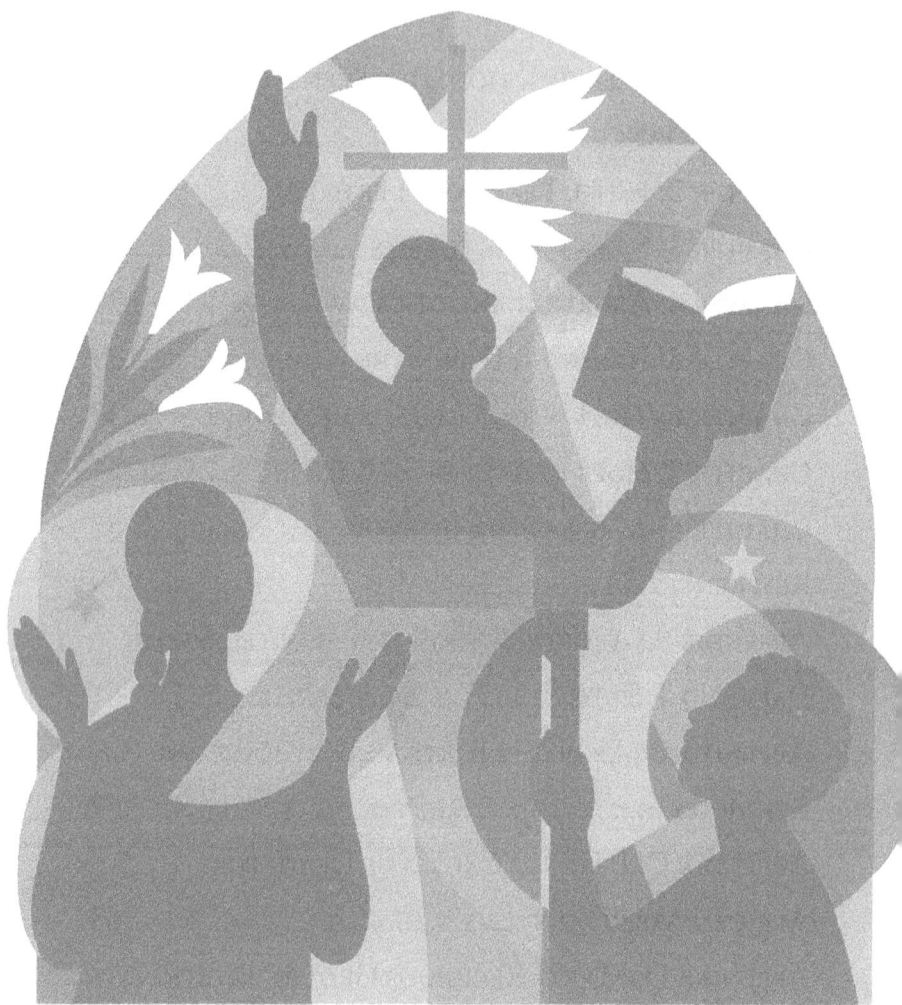

CHAPTER 1

INTRODUCTION: BETWEEN REVERENCE AND RELEVANCE

As I sat in the pew of a worship service at Edgehill United Methodist Church, the air filled with the soft hum of the congregation's murmurs. The guest preacher, Rev. Grace Imathiu, stood confidently at the pulpit, her warm voice reaching every corner of the sanctuary as she shared a memorable story.

She recalled a time when, due to a misprint in the church bulletin, the wrong scripture was read aloud. The assigned reader, unaware of the mix-up, began reading from Genesis 38, the story of Judah and Tamar. The congregation shifted in their seats as the unexpected words filled the space: Jacob's troubling affair with his daughter-in-law. It was meant to be Genesis 28, where Jacob dreams of ascending a ladder toward heaven, a reverent passage many hold dear.

Rev. Imathiu's face flushed slightly as she described the moment. She wasn't prepared to preach from such a controversial text, and yet the misprint had led to a powerful reflection. "I didn't use that passage in my sermon that day," she confessed, a wry smile dancing across her face. "But it got me thinking." Her eyes sparkled with the wisdom of someone who had wrestled with uncomfortable truths.

She explained that Genesis 28, the passage about Jacob's dream, is often viewed as a reverent text—comforting and familiar. It's a scripture that invites the congregation to lean into the divine, with its peaceful, almost ethereal imagery. In contrast, Genesis 38, with its raw and scandalous narrative, might be considered a relevant text—a story that confronts human frailty and sin head-on. Rev. Imathiu paused, allowing the weight of her words to settle in the quiet room.

"Reverence is safe," she continued, her voice steady, yet impassioned, "but relevance is often uncomfortable. It's messy. It's about challenging boundaries, pushing against the familiar, and yes—ruffling some feathers." She glanced around the room, her gaze locking with several members of the congregation. "Most of us prefer the comfort of reverence," she acknowledged, nodding as if in shared understanding. "We don't want to face the complexities, the parts of scripture that expose our weaknesses, our sins, or the parts that ask us to look beyond our neat, tidy boxes of faith."

Her words resonated deeply in the stillness of the room. The light filtered through the stained glass windows, casting multicolored reflections on the pews, as if the sacred space itself was acknowledging the tension between reverence and relevance. Rev. Imathiu went on to elaborate on how the ideal sermon should strike a balance between both: honoring the reverence of tradition while embracing the relevance of truth that challenges us to grow.

As she finished, the sense of unease mingled with inspiration, and I found myself pondering: How often do we shy away from the scriptures that demand something deeper, something rawer? And how often do we choose the safer, more comfortable path of reverence over the sometimes uncomfortable truths of relevance?

During my enrollment in the course, *Feminist and Womanist Theological Ethics*, taught by Vanderbilt Divinity School Professor Stacey Floyd-Thomas, I was required to view the 1996 HBO movie *If These Walls Could Talk*. The film, which portrays the stories of three women facing difficult pregnancies at different points in their lives, sparked an interest in abortion and its many complex issues. The movie provided a backdrop for my final class paper, where I shared the stories of women I interviewed. Though the characters in the film were fictional and White, the five women I interviewed were African-American, and their stories reflected similar struggles with pregnancy during challenging times.

At the same time, I was also completing the second semester of my year-long Field Education internship at Hope Clinic for Women, a non-profit organization in Nashville. The clinic offers a range of services for pregnant women, including counseling, education, and access to necessities like maternity and baby clothes, diapers, and car seats. While the clinic does not perform abortions, many of its clients came in initially considering abortion. This exposure to women grappling with their reproductive choices deepened my interest in the topic and provided a real-world context that informed my understanding of the issues surrounding abortion.

In my final paper for the ethics class titled, "But You Don't Know My Story: A Metaethical Analysis of Abortion from a Womanist Perspective," I chose the following problem:

> We, as Black women who have experienced abortion, have the tendency to remain silent regarding the issue by keeping our experiences to ourselves because we are afraid of the judgmental attitudes others might exhibit toward us. By refusing to speak about our lived realities, due to the fear of appearing "less than," we as African American church goers, have the tendency to deflect any questions regarding our position on the pro-life/ pro-choice debate. Due to different manifestations of shame, we, as female-bodied persons of color …

have the tendency to inhibit possibilities for healing by avoiding those who would ask difficult questions.

The five women I interviewed for my paper came from different phases of my life—two were high school friends, two I knew from college, and one attended my church. Each had her own story, her own struggle, her own moment of decision. Two of the women underwent abortions in the sixties, before the procedure became legal in the United States. One recalled the secrecy, the whispered arrangements, and the fear of discovery. Another, who was married at the time, remembered how her husband held her hand during the initial consultation, his grip both reassuring and uncertain. She described the long 24-hour waiting period before the procedure, how the silence in their home felt heavier than usual, as if the walls themselves were holding their breath. Three of the women had their abortions performed in states outside of Tennessee, each navigating different legal landscapes but all sharing the weight of their choice.

As I wove their stories together with those of the women in *If These Walls Could Talk*, I reached a conclusion that I could no longer ignore: Black women—and men— cannot afford to remain silent about abortion. As members of African-American congregations, we must engage in real, unfiltered conversations about our stance on pro-life and pro-choice issues, along with the broader implications of abortion in our communities. This is not just a political issue—it is deeply personal, spiritual, and generational. With African-American women experiencing abortion at almost four times the rate of White women and nearly twice the rate of Hispanic women, the Black church may be the most crucial place for these discussions to begin.

One of the most pressing contemporary debates on abortion in Tennessee revolved around Amendment 1, a constitutional amendment on the 2014 ballot. The air was thick with tension in the weeks leading up to the vote. Billboards lined the highways, television ads flooded the airwaves, and conversations in grocery store aisles turned political. Tennesseans were asked to decide whether the state legislature should have the authority to regulate abortion. In the days before the election, *The Tennessean* ran a front-page headline in bold, oversized letters: "Amendment 1 Poll: Vote on Abortion 'Too Close to Call.'" The article revealed that, out of 600 registered voters polled, thirty-two percent opposed the amendment, thirty-nine percent supported it, and fifteen percent remained undecided. The rest either refused to answer or did not plan to vote. In the end, the amendment passed, overturning a 2000 Tennessee Supreme Court ruling that had previously protected access to abortion services. Even forty years after *Roe v. Wade*, the battle rages on.

Abortion is a topic that pulls people out of their comfort zones. It is complex, deeply emotional, and often avoided—especially in sacred spaces like the church. But should the church not be both a sacred space and a safe space? Should it not be a place where reverent and relevant sermons, open discussions, and honest testimonies create a foundation for healing and understanding?

My purpose in exploring this difficult subject extends beyond academic curiosity. It is a mission rooted in three goals: (1) to raise awareness of abortion and abortion-related issues, particularly within the Black church; (2) to help individuals clarify their beliefs on the pro-life/pro-choice debate and other legal and ethical questions surrounding abortion; and (3) to equip the Black church with the tools to educate its members and create spaces for honest, faith-centered conversations about abortion and human sexuality as a whole.

Through this process, I hope that those who have experienced abortion will find the courage to share their stories. Their voices matter. Their pain, their choices, and their healing journeys may serve as a beacon for others—whether for women who still carry the weight of guilt, shame, and unresolved grief, or for those who may one day face the same crossroads. Mothers and grandmothers, too, must be part of this conversation, for their daughters and granddaughters may one day need guidance. The silence must end. The conversations must begin. And in that space of dialogue, perhaps, true healing can finally take root.

Should the church play a role in addressing these issues? More specifically, should predominantly Black congregations engage with abortion-related matters, and if so, to what extent?

As a member of a predominantly Black church and denomination, I believe the Black church should be involved. Historically, it has been a foundation for advocacy, guiding both moral and social issues within the community. To explore this further, I will examine historical data, statistical trends, and the perspectives of theologians, feminist scholars, and other relevant voices.

CHAPTER 2

------ ⟫⟫⟩ ⟨⟨⟨⟨ ------

FAITH, FEAR, AND FERTILITY

Amanda had always envisioned a life of devotion. In high school and college, she vowed to remain a virgin, entertaining the thought that she might one day become a nun. Though not Catholic, the idea intrigued her. Maybe she would even be the first Black nun in her community. But life had other plans.

After college, that dream faded into the background, replaced by the distractions of adulthood. On a whim, she spent the night with a man she had dated on and off during her junior and senior years. She cared for him, but they weren't in love. It was brief—"one time only." Over in a minute, she thought. Insignificant. Until it wasn't.

She was pregnant.

Panic gripped her. She had just landed her first teaching job, the start of a career she had worked so hard to achieve. Now, everything felt uncertain. Would she repeat the cycle of her mother—an unwed parent struggling to make ends meet? Would she be forced to live in the projects for the rest of her life? The world was different for women then. In the 1960s and '70s, even married teachers were expected to take a leave of absence or resign once their pregnancies became visible. Staying in the classroom seemed impossible.

Amanda confided in only one person—her closest friend, who worked in a doctor's office known for performing illegal abortions. The decision was made in quiet agony. She severed all ties with the child's father, never telling him about the pregnancy or what she had done. Then, she carried on as if nothing had happened.

Decades passed. She married. Had two children. Built a life. But the past has a way of resurfacing in unexpected ways.

Years later, as she lay on an operating table for a tubal ligation—her choice to ensure she wouldn't have more children—an old fear clawed its way back. What if she was unknowingly pregnant? What if this procedure destroyed another life? The thought burrowed deep, settling into her mind like an unwelcome tenant.

She spiraled. Sleep eluded her. Food lost its taste. Her doctor handed her a prescription for Valium, a small yellow pill promising relief. But as she stared at it in her palm, doubt crept in. Could this really help? Or was this just another way of numbing what she couldn't bring herself to face?

A thought, unshakable and clear, settled in her spirit: The enemy comes to kill, steal, and destroy. She had read the words before, but now they felt alive. Taking the pill would mean surrendering to the despair. Refusing it felt like reclaiming her power. With a deep breath, she set the pill aside and turned to prayer.

Healing didn't come overnight. It came in fragments, in quiet moments of reflection and whispered prayers of repentance. Not just for her fears, but for the choice she had made all those years ago. Back then, she had believed the fetus wasn't truly alive yet. No need to grieve. No need to repent. Just relief at having survived the procedure. But now, she saw things differently.

One night, in the depths of her sorrow, a vision came to her—an image so vivid it felt real. What if, by some miracle, the child she had lost had been transplanted into another woman's womb? The thought, absurd yet strangely comforting, took root. So much so that, for years, she convinced herself that a young woman in her church—who had an unexpected pregnancy shortly after marriage—was, in fact, carrying her child. The mind searches for ways to make peace with the past.

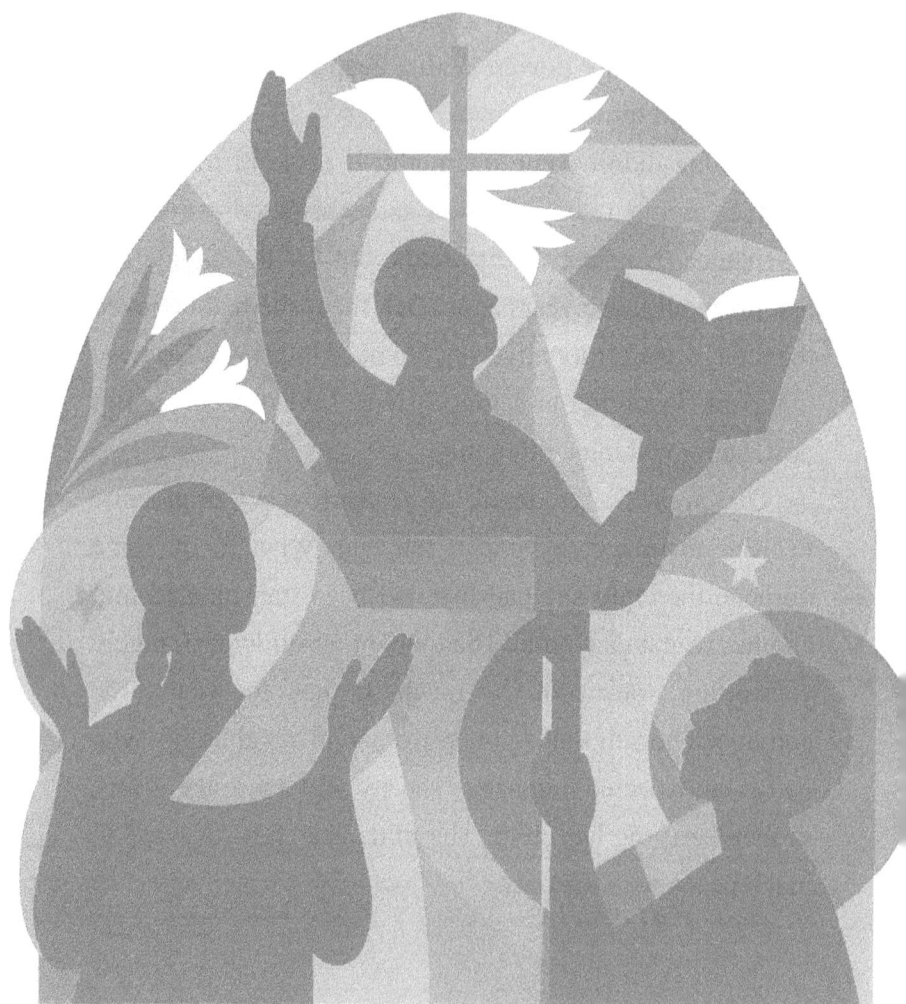

CHAPTER 3

———————⟫⟫⟫ ⟪⟪⟪———————

SILENT SANCTUARIES

Where exactly does the contemporary Christian church stand on this deeply personal, yet politically charged issue? If Amanda had walked into a church before her decision—or even after—what response would she have received?

The answer depends on where she went. The Christian Church remains divided, with differing views among denominations, congregations, and even individuals within the same church. The Roman Catholic Church has stood firm in its opposition to abortion since 1869, when Pope Pius IX declared both contraception and abortion morally unacceptable. Other Christian traditions, however, have taken different stances over time.

In his book *A Love for Life: Christianity's Consistent Protection of the Unborn*, Dennis R. Di Mauro explores how churches have addressed abortion since the 1960s. At one point, the National Council of Churches condemned abortion unless the mother's life was at risk. Yet, as the pro-choice movement gained traction, some denominations pushed for legal reform, even forming the Clergy Consultation Service, a network that secretly referred women to abortion providers abroad.

The Reality of Abortion in the Black Community

African American churches, too, have wrestled with this issue. In 1977, the African Methodist Episcopal Church (AMEC) published a working paper that acknowledged the sanctity of life while making an exception when the mother's life was in danger. Di Mauro shares this passage in his previously mentioned book.

"...The means of relieving the unwanted child of the burden of an undesirable quality of life, or the unwanting parent of the burden of parenthood at an undesirable time, does not lie in the destruction of the new life. Rather, it requires a diligent, active effort, directed by God, to recognize and prevent the circumstances leading to problem pregnancies..."

Meanwhile, the National Baptist Convention, USA, the largest predominantly African American denomination, has no official position on abortion. Each congregation decides how to approach ethical issues like this. In many Black churches, the topic of abortion is often overshadowed by more pressing concerns—racism, education, drug abuse, gang violence—leading to silence rather than outright endorsement or rejection.

Di Mauro suggests that this silence may not reflect indifference, but rather a lack of awareness about how abortion disproportionately affects the Black community.

Although I concur with Di Mauro's conclusion based on his interviews with Black clergy, I believe that silence itself makes a statement (apathy, disbelief, hopelessness, etc.) and that breaking the silence on the issue of abortion serves as the only means of reversing the unfortunate trend that currently exists. In my opinion, breaking the silence represents the first step Black churches can take that might possibly lead to a reduction in the number of abortions experienced by African-American women.

I grew up Baptist—strict, no-nonsense, and full of rules about what was right and wrong. Fornication? Sin. Staying a virgin until marriage? The only acceptable path. Abortion? It wasn't just frowned upon—it simply wasn't discussed. Not at home. Not at church. Not at school. Not even among close friends.

But silence doesn't mean absence.

I remember the woman who lived two doors down. One day, she was fine. The next, an ambulance rushed her away. Whispers floated through the neighborhood. "She tried to do it herself." "Something went wrong." No one said it outright, but we all knew. She had attempted a self-administered abortion, and it had nearly killed her. Still,

21

no one talked about it—not openly. Just murmurs, hushed conversations, and the quiet hope that she'd survive.

Now, decades later, I'm an ordained minister in the African Methodist Episcopal (AME) Church. You'd think things would be different. But the silence remains. Why? Why do so many Black churches avoid this conversation? And why is the abortion rate for African American women still nearly four times higher than that of White women?

These are the questions I seek to explore.

The Guttmacher Institute's 2014 report, consistent with both past and present reports on induced abortions, sheds light on *why* women make this choice:

75% cite financial instability.

75% worry about the impact on work, school, or family responsibilities.

50% fear single parenthood or relationship struggles.

The women I personally interviewed echoed these same concerns. They weren't reckless or indifferent; they were trying to survive. But then, there was the outlier—one woman in a clinic waiting room who casually mentioned she was there for her *fourth* abortion. To her, it was just birth control. No pills. No condoms. Just a quick fix.

Is she the norm? No. But does her story matter? Absolutely.

The Role of Misinformation

Then there's the issue of knowledge—or the lack thereof.

Take Amanda, for example. Like so many others, she wasn't fully aware of fetal development. She hadn't been given the resources, the education, or the support to make a truly informed decision.

How many more women are in Amanda's shoes? How many Black women see abortion as their only option, not because they want to, but because they feel trapped—by finances, by broken relationships, by a system that has failed them?

If the Black church won't talk about abortion, where does that leave the women who are dealing with it?

This isn't about judgment. It's about understanding. It's about confronting the realities that drive these statistics. It's about asking hard questions and pushing past the silence. Because silence doesn't erase the problem—it only ensures that it continues.

Pro-Choice and Pro-Life Debates Over Abortion

The debate over abortion is filled with tough questions and strong emotions. Should abortion be legal? Is the life growing inside the womb a person? Is abortion a religious issue—or even a sin? People on both sides of the debate argue their points passionately, using specific language, personal stories, and even scripture to support their views.

Let's take a look at both perspectives.

The Pro-Choice Argument

According to Stephen Schwartz, a professor emeritus of philosophy and author of *Understanding Abortion*, pro-choice advocates generally believe:

- A woman's quality of life matters, and sometimes abortion is the best decision for her future.

- A fetus is not a person, so terminating a pregnancy is not the same as taking a life.

- Even if the fetus *were* a person, no one should be forced to carry a pregnancy against their will.

For many who support abortion rights, the decision is not about being reckless or careless—it's about having control over their own bodies and futures. Some argue that banning abortion forces women into situations that could be physically, emotionally, or financially harmful.

One woman I spoke to, *Monica*, told me her story. "I was nineteen, working two jobs, barely making rent. When I found out I was pregnant, I panicked. My boyfriend had already left. My mother said, 'You'll figure it out.' But I *knew* I couldn't do it alone. The choice I made was painful, but it was mine."

The Pro-Life Argument

On the other side, pro-life advocates argue:

- The baby in the womb is a living human being.

- Taking an innocent life is morally wrong.

- Abortion is especially horrific because of the violent ways it ends life.

For many, the argument is simple: life begins at conception, and ending that life is wrong. Religious pro-life supporters often turn to scripture. One commonly cited passage is Luke 1:41-44: *"And when Elizabeth heard the greeting of Mary, the baby leaped in her womb."* The idea here is that if John the Baptist could recognize Jesus before birth, then life must begin in the womb.

Both sides claim scripture supports their stance. Interestingly, pro-choice advocates point to passages like Numbers 5, where a husband who suspects his wife of infidelity takes her to a priest, who gives her a bitter drink that can cause miscarriage. Some interpret this as biblical evidence that abortion has a place in certain situations. But the truth is, the Bible doesn't say, "Thou shalt not have an abortion." Unlike clear commandments about murder, lying, or stealing, scripture is largely silent on the topic.

After years of study, reflection, and real-life conversations, I find myself in what some might call a *contradictory* position. Like civil rights activist Fannie Lou Hamer, I believe abortion is a tragedy. She once said, *"The methods used to take human life, such as abortion, the pill, the ring, etc., amount to genocide."* While I wouldn't use the word *genocide*, I do believe in the sanctity of life—both the life of the mother and the unborn child.

Yet, I also know that life isn't always black and white. Some women are trapped in impossible situations, abandoned by their families, struggling to survive. I've listened to their stories. I've seen the pain in their eyes.

I think of Amanda as she whispered, "I don't know what to do. If I have this baby, I lose my job. What does God want me to do?"

As a minister, I don't believe my job is to judge—I believe my job is to *care*.

One article I read, *Can a Christian Be Morally Pro-Life and Politically Pro-Choice?*, argued that a Christian can hold both views for several reasons: personal freedom, justice for women, and the reality that banning abortion doesn't stop it—it just makes it more dangerous.

I get that. I *really* do. That's why if someone asks me, "Are you pro-life or pro-choice?" my answer is simple: *I am both*. I stand for life, but I also stand for compassion, for choice, for the complex reality of human struggle. And I stand for women—no matter what choice they make.

Generally speaking, I believe God is both pro-life and pro-choice. Pro-life because God is the Giver and Sustainer of *all* life, including the unborn. And Pro-Choice because, from the very beginning, when Adam and Eve were placed in the Garden of Eden, God provided them with the opportunity to *choose* by placing the Tree of Knowledge of Good and Evil in the Garden. Think about it. If God had not wanted them to have a choice, then God would have simply *not* placed the tree in the Garden!

CHAPTER 4

————— ❯❯❯❯ ❮❮❮❮ —————

ABORTION AND THE LAW

According to the Centers for Disease Control's 2020 Surveillance Report, abortion is "an intervention performed by a licensed clinician (e.g., a physician, nurse-midwife, nurse practitioner, or physician assistant) that is intended to terminate a suspected or known ongoing intrauterine pregnancy and produce a nonviable fetus at any gestational age." In the United States, abortion law is rooted in constitutional interpretation by the Supreme Court. The Constitution itself does not directly regulate abortion; rather, it sets limits on how states and the federal government can regulate it.

America's stance on abortion has shifted dramatically over the years. In the early 19th century, abortion was widely accessible, often performed without medical oversight. Women could even induce them on their own. Historian Dorothy McBride explains, "Anybody could and did use all manner of means to end pregnancies... because of the law that reinforced the doctrine that abortions before quickening were not killing a human being but solving a female problem."

But as medicine advanced, so did scrutiny over abortion. In 1847, the American Medical Association (AMA) was formed, aiming to professionalize the medical field. By 1859, the AMA had declared that abortion at any stage was the killing of a human being and called for its criminalization, except when necessary to save a woman's life. Physicians argued that women sought abortions due to ignorance of fetal development—an ignorance they saw as their duty to correct.

This tightening grip on abortion laws played out over the decades. In 1821, Connecticut passed the first abortion statute, criminalizing the use of poison to induce abortion after quickening. Other states soon followed. By 1840, ten of the twenty-six states had enacted abortion restrictions. The AMA's influence grew, and by 1900, every state had criminalized abortion, with only rare exceptions.

Meanwhile, religious opposition to abortion was mounting. In 1869, Pope Pius IX officially condemned abortion and contraception, declaring that life began at conception. Four years later, Congress passed the Comstock Act, making it a federal crime to distribute information about contraception or abortion. This wave of restrictions lasted for decades, driving abortion underground.

But as the 20th century progressed, the conversation around reproductive rights began to shift. In 1916, Margaret Sanger opened the first birth control clinic in America. She was soon jailed for violating the Comstock Act, but her activism laid the foundation for what would become Planned Parenthood. By the 1950s and 60s, medical advancements and shifting cultural attitudes spurred calls for abortion law reform. In 1959, the American Law Institute proposed a model law allowing abortion in cases of rape, incest, fetal deformity, or threats to the mother's health. By 1970, Hawaii became the first state to legalize abortion in the first twenty weeks of pregnancy.

Then, in 1973, everything changed. The Supreme Court's landmark Roe v. Wade decision struck down state bans on abortion, ruling that a woman's right to choose was protected under the constitutional right to privacy. The ruling divided the nation, fueling the rise of the pro-life and pro-choice movements. The March for Life was first organized in 1974, while abortion rights activists continued pushing for expanded access.

Throughout the following decades, the legal and political battles continued. In 1986, the National Organization for Women (NOW) and other feminist organizations led the first national March for Women's Lives, bringing over 100,000 advocates to Washington, D.C.

In 2016 the Supreme Court made a ruling on the Whole Woman's Health v. Hellerstedt case, dictating that Texas could not place restrictions on abortion services that create an undue burden for women seeking an abortion. Then, six years later, on June 24, 2022, the Supreme court overturned Roe v. Wade, leaving abortion decisions up to states and no longer a constitutional right. Today, abortion remains one of the most polarizing issues in America. In recent years, states have passed laws either expanding or restricting access.

Take parental notification and consent laws. Imagine a sixteen-year-old girl, sitting across from a doctor, hands clenched together, heart pounding. The doctor explains that in her state, she cannot get an abortion without a parent's permission. She knows her mother, a devout Christian, would never agree. Pro-life advocates believe parents should have a say in such a major decision. Pro-choice activists counter that these laws violate a young woman's right to privacy and could force vulnerable girls into unsafe situations.

Then there's mandated counseling. Picture a woman sitting in a clinic, listening to a health professional read from a state-mandated script about fetal development and abortion alternatives. But according to a 2025 report by the Guttmacher Institute, twenty-three states require individuals to receive counseling and to then wait for a period of time before getting an abortion. Intended to deter patients, 14 states require in-person counseling and 6 states make patients wait 72 hours before they can receive their abortion.

In 1992, the Supreme Court weighed in through *Planned Parenthood v. Casey*, reviewing Pennsylvania's strict abortion law. The law required a 24-hour waiting period, parental consent, and spousal notification. In a splintered decision, the Court upheld the waiting period and parental consent but struck down the spousal notification requirement, reinforcing that a woman's autonomy could not be entirely overridden by state mandates.

Currently, abortions are illegal in 13 states. Women faced with unwanted pregnancies in any of these 13 states must travel outside their state if they choose abortion as an option. In several states, because of their strict laws, all abortions, including medication abortions, are prohibited, even for rape and incest, and can be performed only when the mother's life is in danger.

According to the Knoxville News Sentinel in June 2024, "two years after overturning the constitutional right to an abortion, the Supreme Court went the other direction and tossed out a challenge to mifepristone, a drug used to end a pregnancy that is less than 70 days developed, that would have curbed access to the drug and jeopardized the independence of the Food and Drug Administration."

The fight over abortion rights is far from settled. As in times past, America continues to wrestle with the question: Should women have the right to choose?

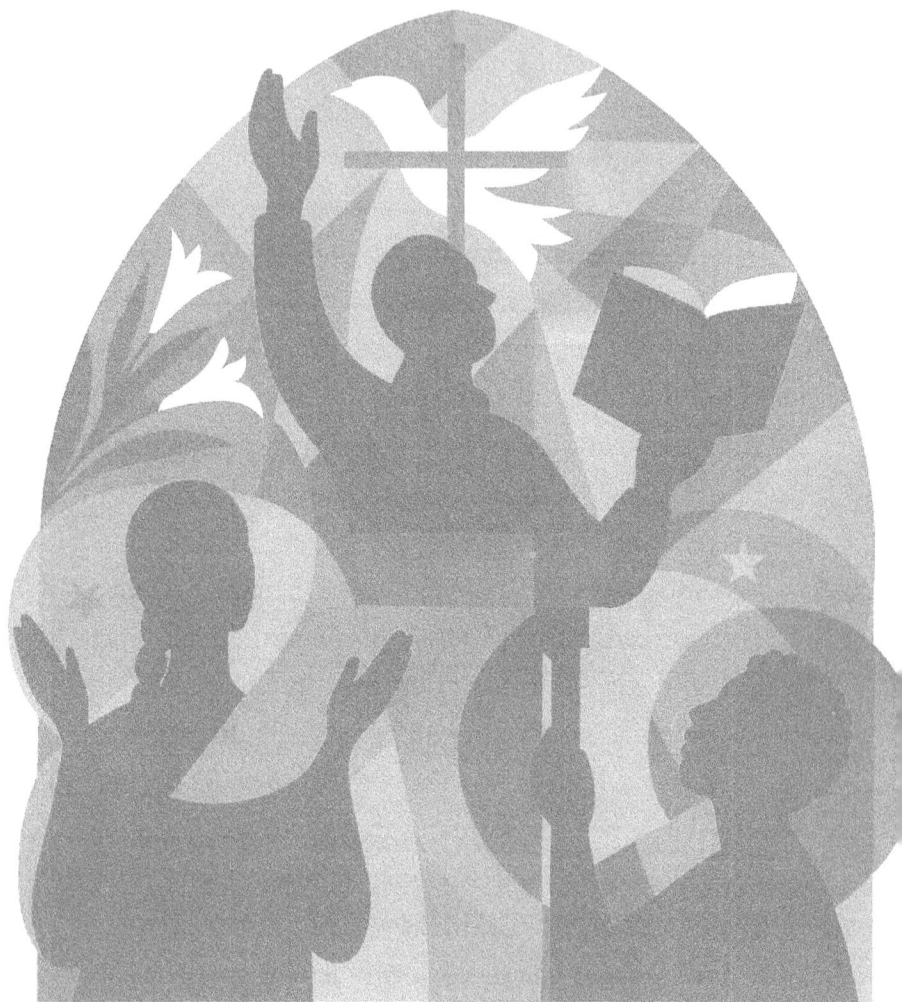

CHAPTER 5

———— »»»› ‹‹‹«« ————

BREAKING DOWN THE NUMBERS

One in four women in the United States will have an abortion by age 45. Between 1973 and 2022, the beginning and end of Roe v. Wade, the total number of abortions in America is estimated at 64,443,118.

The debate over abortion is often framed by statistics. According to the most recent United States Abortion Surveillance Report from the Centers for Disease Control and Prevention (CDC), data were collected from 49 of the 52 reporting areas, which include the 50 states, the District of Columbia, and New York City. In 2020 alone, a total of 765,651 abortions were reported. The report also provided a demographic breakdown: among the 38 areas that reported marital status, 85.3% of women who obtained abortions were unmarried, while 14.7% were married. In terms of previous abortions, 55.4% of women reported having none, while 36.1% had undergone one or two, and 8.5% had three or more.

The landscape of abortion services has also evolved. According to the Guttmacher Institute, in 2011, 59% of abortion providers—about 1,023 facilities nationwide—offered early medication abortions following the FDA's approval of mifepristone as an alternative to surgical procedures. That same year, medication abortions accounted for 23% of all nonhospital abortions and 36% of abortions performed before nine weeks of gestation.

Throughout history, women of all ages, ethnicities, religious backgrounds, and socioeconomic statuses have sought abortions. The 2020 CDC Abortion Surveillance Report estimated that approximately 1.2 million abortions were performed annually in the United States. Meanwhile, the Guttmacher Institute reported that between 1973—when abortion was legalized—and 2011, nearly 53 million legal abortions took place.

Additional findings from the 2020 CDC report include:

- Women in their 20s accounted for the majority of abortions (57.2%), while those under 15 and over 40 represented the smallest percentages (0.2% and 3.7%, respectively).

- Non-Hispanic White and Black women had the highest percentages of abortions (32.7% and 39.2%, respectively), while Hispanic women and women of other races accounted for 21.1% and 7.0%.

- Non-Hispanic White women had the lowest abortion rate (6.2 abortions per 1,000 women aged 15-44), whereas Non-Hispanic Black women had the highest (24.4 abortions per 1,000 women aged 15-44).

The statistics are hard to ignore. According to the 2020 Centers for Disease Control (CDC) Surveillance Report, the abortion rate for non-Hispanic Black women was 3.9 times higher than for non-Hispanic White women and more than twice as high as for Hispanic women. But numbers only tell part of the story.

These statistics highlight a significant disparity: while White and Black women have nearly equal percentages of total abortions, the abortion rate for Black women is almost four times higher. This stark contrast underscores the higher rate of unintended pregnancies among Black women—a disparity that has been a major factor in my decision to explore this issue further.

According to a 2021 report by Human Life Initiative, the leading causes of death for African Americans – Heart Disease (90,507); Cancer (70,036); COVID (55,994); Accidents (33,830); Drug Induced (19,212); Diabetes (18,968); and homicides (14,313) – were greatly outnumbered by Abortions (262,911).

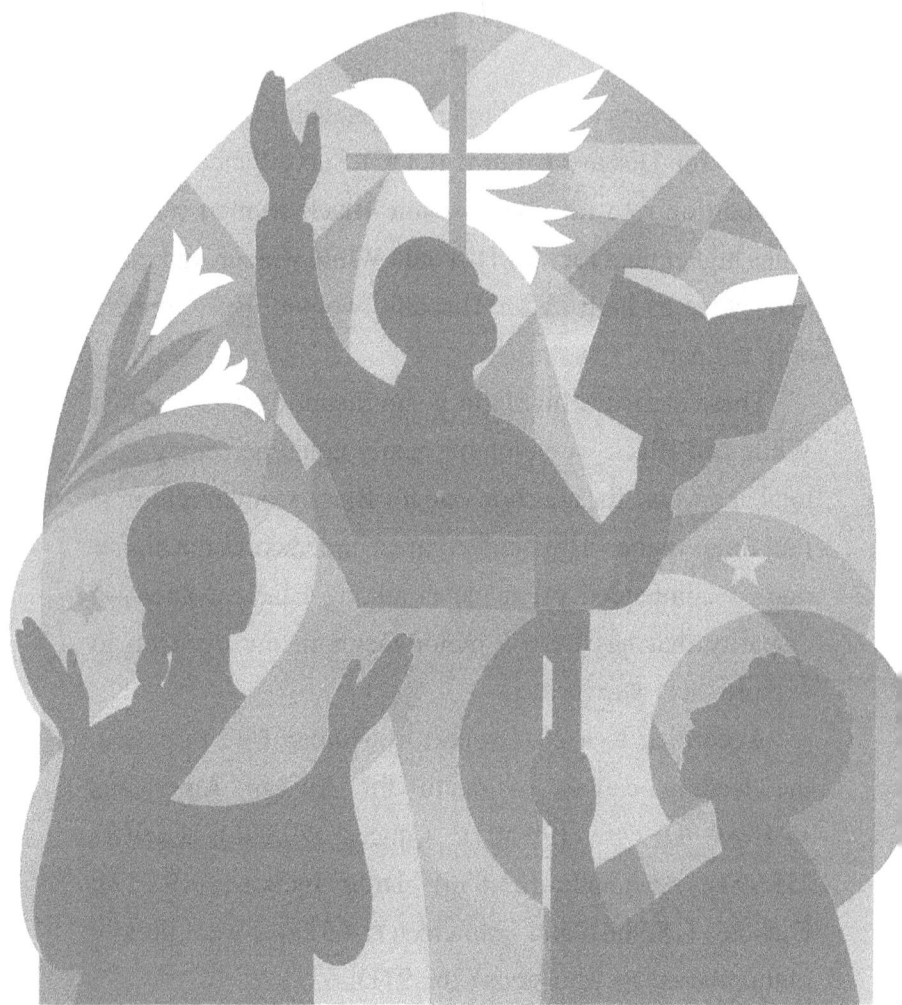

CHAPTER 6

THE UNTOLD LEGACY OF ABORTION AMONG BLACK WOMEN

For African Americans, the history of abortion is deeply intertwined with slavery. Enslaved Black women, treated as property, were expected to reproduce for the economic benefit of their owners. But they resisted.

In *Black Woman's Burden*, sociologist Nicole Rousseau recounts a chilling historical account: A plantation owner, puzzled by the low birth rate among his enslaved women, discovered that they had concocted a medicine to terminate pregnancies. Another master lamented that an older female slave had developed a remedy that "was instrumental in all the abortions on his place."

"There were many ways enslaved women resisted," Rousseau writes, "and refusing to bring children into bondage was one of them."

Historian Loretta J. Ross, in her article "African-American Women and Abortion: 1880-1970," describes how methods ranged from herbal medicines to strenuous labor and even physical trauma. Though records are sparse, Ross emphasizes that the significance lies not in how frequently these acts occurred but in the fact that they happened at all.

Rousseau captures the emotional turmoil of these women: "The enslaved Black woman sees her power, even in her oppressed state. She understands that the system depends on her body to function. When she has no other choice, she takes the only meaningful action left. She carries the pain of her decision and continues to survive."

For the enslaved women, speaking about their experiences would have carried dire consequences—not just for themselves but for anyone connected to the act. Silence was survival. If shame accompanied the experience, silence became a way to bury the memory, to push it deep enough that it wouldn't surface again.

And so began the silence. This silence has echoed through generations. Black women, raised in households where "What happens in this house stays in this house" was the rule, learned to keep their pain locked away. Of the five women I interviewed for my first book, *But...You Don't Know My Story,* four had never spoken of their abortion experience before. They had absorbed the same unspoken message: certain things were never to be discussed. Even now, the weight of that silence lingers.

Today, many women who have had abortions remain silent for similar reasons. Fear of judgment, condemnation, and the resurfacing of emotions—shame, regret, or even relief—keeps them quiet. Some worry about being ostracized by their communities, particularly in religious settings. Others choose silence because they feel there is no space where they can speak freely without consequence.

But what happens when silence breaks?

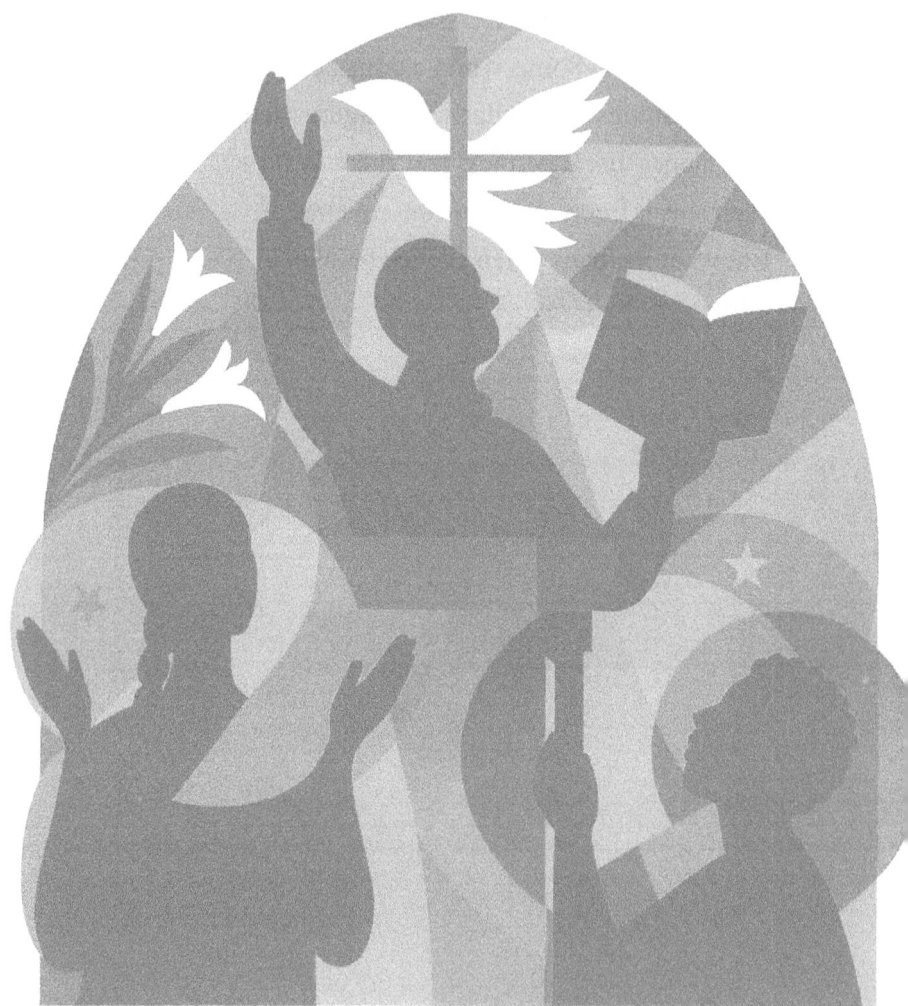

CHAPTER 7

HOPE IN ACTION:
STRATEGIC SOLUTIONS FOR THE
BLACK CHURCH AND ABORTION

The debate over abortion is relentless. It flares up in political arenas, on social media, and in the pews of churches. But amid all the noise, the most critical question remains: where are these conversations really happening? Are mothers sitting down with their daughters, whispering hard truths over kitchen tables? Are church leaders stepping out from behind their pulpits to listen, really listen, to the struggles of their congregants? Are women who have walked the path of abortion reaching out to those who stand at the crossroads, uncertain and afraid?

According to the most recent Abortion Surveillance Report by the Centers for Disease Control and Prevention (CDC):

"Multiple factors are known to influence the incidence of abortion, including the availability of abortion providers; state regulations such as mandatory waiting periods, parental involvement laws, and legal restrictions on abortion providers; increasing acceptance of non-marital childrearing; shifts in the racial/ethnic composition of the U.S. population; and changes in the economy and resulting impact on fertility preferences and access to health-care services, including contraception. However, despite these multiple influences, given that unintended pregnancy precedes nearly all abortions, efforts to reduce the incidence of abortion need to focus on helping women avoid pregnancies that they do not desire."

The takeaway is clear: preventing unwanted pregnancies is key. But prevention isn't just about access to birth control or sex education; it's about community, relationships, and the support systems that shape a woman's choices long before she finds herself staring at a positive pregnancy test.

Marie Costa, author of *Abortion: Contemporary World Issues*, opens her book with a powerful statement: "Abortion, a word once rarely spoken out loud, has over the last three decades become synonymous with controversy and conflict." While that may be true on a public level, abortion still remains an unspoken secret in many Black households. It's a conversation whispered about but never addressed head-on. And until families, churches, and schools have open, honest discussions about abortion—not just its legality but its emotional, spiritual, and societal implications—nothing will change. Silence will continue to breed fear, and fear will continue to drive desperate decisions.

Frederica Mathewes-Green, a researcher on abortion issues, found that many women who choose abortion do so because they feel unsupported. If a woman cannot find love, encouragement, and guidance from her parents, partner, or community, she often believes she has no other option. This is why support must be both vocal and actionable. Compassion isn't just a feeling; it's an action. When Christians come together to offer real, tangible help—whether through mentorship, financial aid, or simply listening without judgment—they embody the teachings of Christ in a way that legislation never could.

Recently, media outlets have been flooded with opinion pieces on abortion from lawyers, doctors, politicians, parents, and clergy. This surge in discussion presents a powerful opportunity. The media can be more than just a battleground for ideological warfare; it can be a bridge to real, meaningful conversations. It can be a tool to educate, to challenge, and most importantly, to engage people on a personal level.

So, how do we turn discussion into action? Below are strategic practices that can be implemented in various settings to foster deeper dialogue, provide education, and ultimately empower individuals to make informed, values-driven decisions regarding abortion:

1. **Community Conversations** - Churches, schools, and community centers should host open forums where individuals can share their experiences and concerns about abortion in a judgment-free environment.

2. **Mentorship Programs** - Women who have faced unplanned pregnancies should be encouraged to mentor young women, offering firsthand insight and emotional support.

3. **Church Engagement** - Rather than preaching condemnation, churches can provide tangible support for single mothers and at-risk youth, helping them see alternative options to abortion.

4. **Educational Workshops** - Schools should integrate discussions on relationships, decision-making, and the emotional and spiritual aspects of pregnancy into their curricula, equipping students with both knowledge and perspective.

5. **Media Utilization** - Instead of allowing media to fuel political division, churches and organizations should use platforms like blogs, podcasts, and social media to spread stories of hope, resilience, and practical support.

6. **Legislative Advocacy** - Those passionate about pro-life efforts should focus on policies that support maternal health, affordable childcare, and economic resources for struggling families—solutions that address the root causes of abortion rather than just its symptoms.

7. **Community Outreach**– Human Life Alliance, which has served the pro-life community around the world for more than 46 years, includes in its abortion-related goals to "Reach Students on Every Campus Every Year." Certainly, reaching out to students on college campuses serves as another means of improving and enhancing communication about abortion and its related issues.

The bottom line? People need to talk. But more than that, they need to act. No law or political argument will ever replace the power of a caring hand, a listening ear, and a heart willing to walk alongside someone in crisis. The silence surrounding abortion has lasted long enough. It's time to break it.

Conversations During Clergy-Led Conferences

In Ohio, a *Choose Life Conference* brought together pastors and community leaders to address what they called "a war on Black babies, a war on Black women, and a war on Black families." As reported by the *Beacon Journal*, during the conference, Star Parker, founder for the Center for Urban Renewal and Education (CURE), shared her personal experience. She stood before the crowd, her voice steady yet passionate. "I was once one of those statistics," she admitted. "But now, I use my story to help others rethink their choices."

The room fell silent, the weight of her words settling over the audience. She continued, "Abortion is deeply embedded in our community, and we have to be outraged. The work of the body of Christ is not being done, particularly in the Black community... This may be legal, but it is not lawful in God's eyes."

Conferences like these provide a space for meaningful conversations. When clergy and laypersons engage in open dialogue, they foster understanding and create pathways for change.

Conversations Through Clergy-Led Lobbying

In Washington, D.C., a group of African-American clergy gathered on Capitol Hill, demanding a congressional investigation into the abortion industry. Pastor Stephen Broden of Fair Park Bible Fellowship in Dallas took the podium. "The church has hesitated on this issue for too long," he declared. "In an attempt to be politically correct, we've avoided the hard conversations. But the majority of our community is buying into an ideology that contradicts the biblical value of life."

His words stirred the crowd. Some nodded in agreement, while others furrowed their brows in contemplation. These clergy members had taken their convictions beyond the pulpit, using their voices to influence policy. Whether pro-life or pro-choice, ministers must engage in these discussions, not to push an agenda, but to serve their congregations with wisdom and compassion.

Conversations Involving Public Policy

Should Christians advocate for public policies related to abortion? And if so, how?

States like Tennessee have introduced regulations to discourage or restrict abortion—waiting periods, parental consent laws, mandatory ultrasounds, and educational materials on fetal development. Some Christians see these laws as necessary measures to uphold the sanctity of life, while others view them as barriers that disproportionately affect marginalized women.

Dr. Willie Parker, a former medical director for Planned Parenthood, sees his work differently. In an interview with *Esquire*, he described his decision to leave a prestigious career to become an abortion provider. "My belief in God tells me that the most important thing you can do for another human being is help them in their time of need," he said.

His words challenge the narrative. For some, he is a hero; for others, a villain. But regardless of where one stands, his story forces us to ask hard questions about faith, ethics, and public policy.

Public policy strategies suggested by ethicist Glen Stassen include:

• Expanding access to non-abortive contraceptives

- Combating sexual violence, including rape and incest
- Promoting sexual responsibility for both men and women
- Increasing availability of high-quality, affordable daycare
- Encouraging business practices that support work-life balance
- Including sterilization and contraceptives in insurance coverage
- Addressing poverty, which often contributes to unplanned pregnancies
- Improving adoption services and reforming adoption laws
- Strengthening support systems for pregnant women and new mothers

Stassen emphasizes that change is possible. "We are not without hope," he writes. "Steadfast initiatives can and do make a difference."

And isn't that what this conversation is ultimately about? Hope. Hope that open dialogue can lead to understanding. Hope that practical strategies can provide alternatives. Hope that communities—families, churches, and policymakers—can come together to create a future where fewer women feel forced to make an impossible choice.

Conversations within Church Settings

The conversation began with a simple question: "How many of you have heard about Amendment 1?" I scanned the room, watching as hands hesitantly lifted, some uncertain, some eager to share their opinions. The women's Bible study group, a mixed-gender Bible study group, and the intercessory prayer team—three distinct groups within my church—had gathered to discuss an issue that had been splashed across newspaper headlines and television ads for weeks.

I had brought in two editorials from *The Tennessean*, published just days earlier. One article, *A No Vote on 1 Averts Threat to Women's Health*, made a strong case for reproductive rights. The other, *Voting Yes on 1 Is the Christian Thing to Do*, urged believers to consider their faith when heading to the polls. I handed copies to each person, allowing time for them to read. The room fell silent except for the rustling of paper and the occasional murmur of contemplation.

Then the discussion took off. Some spoke passionately about their personal convictions, while others wrestled with conflicting emotions, grateful for the opportunity to voice concerns in a setting that welcomed open dialogue. By the end, several members approached me, expressing gratitude. "No one ever talks about these things in church," one woman confided. "I've always had questions, but I never felt comfortable bringing them up."

Moments like these reaffirmed my belief that such conversations belong in churches—especially in predominately Black congregations, where open discussions about sexuality, reproductive health, and controversial social issues are often avoided. The church should be a place where people come for guidance, not just doctrine, and certainly not silence.

Conversations within Church-Sponsored After-School Programs

Later that week, I took the same approach with a different audience: the 14-to-18-year-olds in my church's after-school program. Their response was just as striking. Though too young to vote, they eagerly engaged with the topic, sharing their thoughts on the amendment and what it could mean for their futures.

"So, if this passes, does that mean people will have fewer rights?" one girl asked.

"It depends on how you look at it," I said. "Some believe it protects unborn life. Others believe it restricts women's choices. That's why it's important to be informed and think critically about these issues."

The staff and volunteers chimed in, encouraging the teens to take the discussion home and talk to their parents about the upcoming vote. Some of the youth shared stories— relatives, friends, and classmates who had been affected by abortion in one way or another. These conversations weren't just theoretical debates; they were deeply personal.

What struck me most was their openness. No one shied away from asking hard questions. No one dismissed another's experience. If we want to shape future leaders who think critically about social issues, we need to create more spaces like this—multi-generational dialogues where wisdom meets curiosity, and where young people feel heard rather than lectured.

Conversations Led by Outside Groups

My journey through these conversations didn't stop within the walls of the church. As part of my Master of Divinity program, I spent a year interning at Hope Clinic for Women, a non-profit that provides care and counseling for pregnant women. The clinic takes a pro-life stance but also offers education and prevention programs to schools, churches, and community organizations.

One day, I sat in on a session led by the clinic's education and prevention specialist at a community center in a low-income neighborhood. The audience: a group of middle school students. The topic: pregnancy prevention, pornography, and abortion. The room buzzed with energy as kids asked raw, unfiltered questions. The specialist didn't shy away from answering.

Later, I attended another session—this time in an affluent neighborhood, where a group of homeschooling mothers gathered at a large interdenominational church. The discussion had a different tone, more measured, more policy-focused, but no less engaged. It was clear that the need for these conversations spanned all demographics, cutting across socioeconomic and cultural lines.

Following my internship, I was invited to join the Hope Clinic's Board of Directors. In that role, I saw firsthand how critical these discussions were—not just for those facing unplanned pregnancies, but for communities as a whole. Whether in a church, a school, or a community center, these conversations had the power to inform, challenge, and inspire action.

Churches, schools, and community organizations should take note. We need to seek out partnerships with groups that are willing to facilitate open and honest discussions about these issues. Because at the heart of it all, these are not just debates. They are stories. They are lives.

And they deserve to be heard.

Conversations via Shared Storytelling

Exhale, an online community for individuals seeking to share their abortion experiences as a means of support and advocacy, describes itself as a "pro-voice" space. It is a community filled with people who have had abortions and those who care deeply about individuals with personal abortion experiences. According to the Exhale website:

> "...we support each other by listening without judgment, by sharing our experiences of healing and well-being after abortion, and by finding creative ways to reach out and send the message that our community welcomes new members with love and respect... with the hope of inspiring more advocates

to consider our community members as experts and partners whose contributions can strengthen any advocacy agenda."

The platform invites advocates working on abortion issues to share their personal stories, offering a training guide to help individuals become effective storytellers. This space serves as a source of information and inspiration for those facing difficult choices related to abortion, ensuring that no one feels alone in their journey.

Similarly, Hope Clinic for Women provides an opportunity for its clients to share their personal stories, though from a different perspective. Many women initially visit the clinic considering abortion but ultimately decide to carry their pregnancy to term. These women are invited to share their experiences for publication in one of the clinic's brochures, reinforcing the power of storytelling as a means of connection and support for those navigating complex emotions and decisions.

Conversations in Pastoral Care Spaces

For many, the church is a place of refuge, a space where they seek guidance in moments of crisis—including pre- or post-abortion experiences. Pastoral care and counseling play a crucial role in addressing these deeply personal matters. Clergy must be proactive in creating safe, nonjudgmental spaces where parishioners can share their struggles.

Pastors should clearly communicate the types of support available under the umbrella of pastoral care and ensure that individuals are aware of confidentiality protections in their state. In addition to offering spiritual guidance, clergy should familiarize themselves with external resources, such as counseling services and crisis pregnancy support, so they can provide informed referrals when necessary.

Conversations from the Pulpit

Abortion remains one of the most delicate and controversial topics within church settings, rarely addressed from the pulpit. However, preaching and teaching on the subject—framed within the context of sin, forgiveness, restoration, and reconciliation—can provide clarity, healing, and hope. As theologian Glen Stassen suggests, "Christian leaders should in their teaching and preaching present the best case they can for their perspective..." while also offering tangible support for women facing crisis pregnancies.

I recall a sermon I delivered at my home church where I shared my own abortion experience as a testimony of God's grace, forgiveness, and unwavering love. I imagine some people thought I had revealed too much, but after the service, several individuals approached me, expressing gratitude for my openness. They felt seen, understood, and less alone. Given that one in four women has experienced an abortion, I am certain my testimony resonated with more people than those who spoke up that day.

As an ordained minister in the African Methodist Episcopal (AME) Church, I intend to use the knowledge gained from this journey to reach beyond the walls of my congregation. Whether through pastoral care, counseling, teaching, preaching, or prayer, I am committed to making a difference in the lives of those affected by abortion. I remain hopeful—hopeful that the number of abortions in our country will decline, hopeful that churches, particularly Black churches, will play a pivotal role in providing support, and hopeful that more people will have the courage to break the silence surrounding this issue.

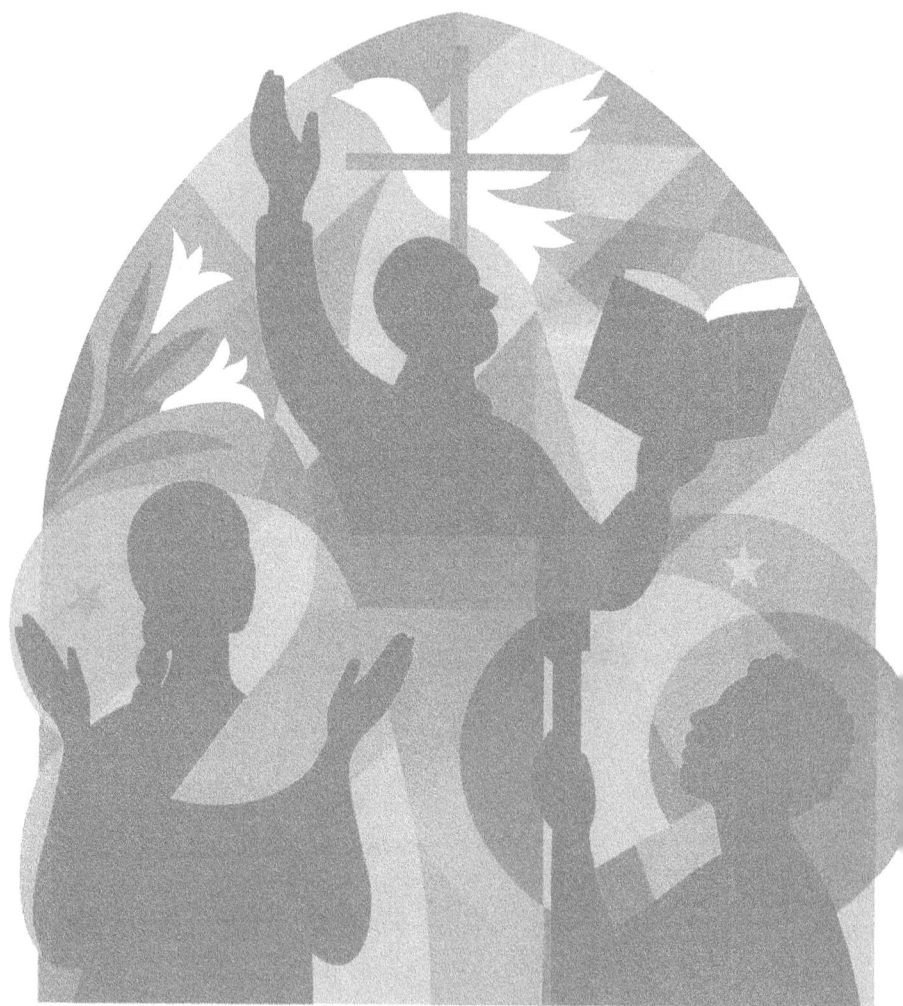

CHAPTER 8

A VISION FOR CHANGE

Education is key. Conversations are critical. Action is necessary. By promoting comprehensive education on abortion, advocating for effective contraception, and fostering open discussions, we can create meaningful change.

Imagine if pro-life and pro-choice advocates set aside their differences and collaborated to reduce the number of abortions rather than advancing opposing agendas. What if the African Methodist Episcopal Church—the oldest Black denomination—joined forces with the National Baptist Convention, USA—the largest Black denomination—to address unintended pregnancies within the Black community? What if their advocacy led to actionable programs and resources within their congregations, resulting in a measurable decline in abortion rates?

What if American's focus shifted from pro-life/pro-choice debates to a discussion that gets to the core of the problem—the prevention of unwanted pregnancies—launching a nation-wide pro-prevention movement? The possibilities give me hope.

And so, with tear-filled but joyful eyes, I conclude this reflection by thinking of Amanda, a young woman whose story I shared earlier. Her experience echoes the words of Dr. Willie Parker, who once said in an *Esquire* article:

"I see women who are crying because they are Christians and they are torn up by the fact that they don't believe in abortion but they're about to have one. What I tell them is that doesn't make you a hypocrite. You can never say what you will do until you're in the situation, and Christians get in jacked-up situations, too."

If Amanda were here, I believe she would nod and say, "I totally get it."

The conversation must continue.

REFERENCES

Centers for Disease Control and Prevention (CDC). (2020). Abortion Surveillance — United States, 2019. https://www.cdc.gov/reproductivehealth/data_stats/abortion.htm

Di Mauro, D. R. (2007). A Love for Life: Christianity's Consistent Protection of the Unborn. Wipf and Stock Publishers.

Esquire. (2015). Dr. Willie Parker on Why He Performs Abortions. https://www.esquire.com/news-politics/a36228/abortion-doctor-willie-parker-interview/

Feinberg, A. (2024, June 14). Supreme Court upholds access to mifepristone: What the abortion pill ruling means in Tennessee. *Knoxville News Sentinel.*

Floyd-Thomas, S. (2013). Feminist and Womanist Theological Ethics. Vanderbilt University Course Material.

Guttmacher Institute. (2020). Abortion Incidence and Service Availability in the United States. https://www.guttmacher.org/

Human Life Initiative. (2021). Leading Causes of Death in the African-American Community.

Jenkins, Colette, *Boston Journal*, August 12, 2012

Mathewes-Green, F. (2004). Real Choices: Listening to Women, Looking for Alternatives to Abortion. Conciliar Press.

McBride, D. (1999). Abortion in the United States: A Reference Handbook. ABC-CLIO.

Pope Pius IX. (1869). Papal Decree on Abortion and Contraception.

Ross, L. J. (1993). African-American Women and Abortion: 1880–1970. In Policing the National Body: Sex, Race, and Criminalization.

Rousseau, N. (2006). Black Woman's Burden: Commodifying Black Reproduction. Lexington Books.

Schwartz, S. (2011). Understanding Abortion: From Mixed Feelings to Rational Thought. Lexington Books.

Stassen, G. (2003). Just Peacemaking: Transforming Initiatives for Justice and Peace. Westminster John Knox Press.

The Tennessean. (2014). Amendment 1 Poll: Vote on Abortion 'Too Close to Call.'

Reported Annual Abortions

	Guttmacher	CDC	
1973	744,610	615,831	
1974	898,570	763,476	
1975	1,034,170	854,853	
1976	1,179,300	988,267	
1977	1,316,700	1,079,430	
1978	1,409,600	1,157,776	
1979	1,497,670	1,251,921	
1980	1,553,890	1,297,606	
1981	1,577,340	1,300,760	
1982	1,573,920	1,303,980	
1983	1,575,000	1,268,987	
1984	1,577,180	1,333,521	
1985	1,588,550	1,328,570	
1986	1,574,000	1,328,112	
1987	1,559,110	1,353,671	
1988	1,590,750	1,371,285	
1989	1,566,900	1,396,658	
1990	1,608,600	1,429,247	
1991	1,556,510	1,388,937	
1992	1,528,930	1,359,146	
1993	1,495,000	1,330,414	
1994	1,423,000	1,267,415	
1995	1,359,400	1,210,883	
1996	1,360,160	1,225,937	
1997	1,335,000	1,186,039	
1998	1,319,000	884,273*	
1999	1,314,800	861,789*	
2000	1,312,990	857,475*	
2001	1,291,000	853,485*	
2002	1,269,000	854,122*	
2003	1,250,000	848,163*	
2004	1,222,100	839,226*	
2005	1,206,200	820,151*	
2006	1,242,200	852,385*	
2007	1,209,640	827,609*	
2008	1,212,350	825,564*	
2009	1,151,600	789,217*	
2010	1,102,670	765,651*	
2011	1,058,490	730,322*	
2012	1,011,000	699,202*	
2013	958,700	664,435*	
2014	926,190	652,639*	
2015	899,500	638,169*	
2016	874,100	623,471*	
2017	862,320	612,719*	
2018	885,800	619,591*	*Excludes NH, CA and often
2019	916,640	629,898*	at least one
2020	930,160	620,327*	other state.
2021	930,160 §		§ NRLC
2022	900,414 §		projection for calculation

ABORTION STATISTICS
United States Data and Trends

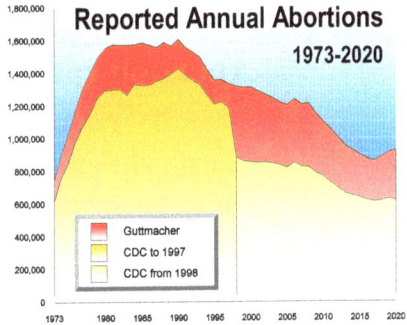

Reported Annual Abortions
1973-2020

There are two basic sources on abortion data in the U.S.:
- The U.S. Centers for Disease Control (CDC) publishes yearly, but relies on voluntary reports from state health departments (and New York City, Washington, D.C.). It has been missing data from California, New Hampshire, and at least one other state since 1998.
- The Guttmacher Institute (GI) contacts abortion clinics directly for data but does not always survey every year.
- Because it surveys clinics directly and includes data from all fifty states, most re-searchers believe Guttmacher's numbers to be more reliable, though Guttmacher still believes it may miss some abortions.

While both Guttmacher and the CDC show big drops over the last 30 years, recent years show increases.
- Total abortions dropped 29.8% from 1998 to 2020 with the CDC, and fell 42.2% from 1990 to 2020 with GI.
- The **abortion rate** for 2020 for GI was 14.4 abortions for every 1,000 women of re-productive age (15-44), less than half that of the high of 29.3 in 1981. While up since 2017 (13.5), it is still lower than when abortion was legalized in the U.S. in 1973 (16.3).
- GI says there were 20.6 abortions for every 100 pregnancies ending in live birth or abortion in 2020, up from 18.3 in 2016, the lowest **abortion ratio** since 1972.
- GI says that abortion "providers" rose slightly to 1,603 in 2020 from 1,587 in 2017. The high was 2,918 in 1982.
- According to the GI, more than half (53%) of abortions were done with chemical abortifacients like mifepristone in 2020. It had been just 16.4% as recently as 2008.
- In June 2022, *Dobbs* overturned *Roe*, activating "trigger laws" in some states offering the unborn full protection or otherwise limiting abortion. Many clinics closed, but some women went to other states or ordered abortion pills online.

The Consequences of *Roe v. Wade*

64,443,118

Total abortions since 1973

Based on numbers reported by the Guttmacher Institute 1973-2020, with 3% added for GI estimated possible 3-5% undercount for 1973-2014. Additional 12,000 per year for 2015-2017 for abortions from "providers" GI says it may have missed in 2015-2017 counts. 2022 estimate projects drops from states with trigger laws since *Dobbs*. 01/23

61

GUTTMACHER INSTITUTE

Abortion rates continue to vary
by race and ethnicity

Lack of access to health insurance and health care plays a
role, as do racism and discrimination

Abortions per 1,000 women aged 15-44

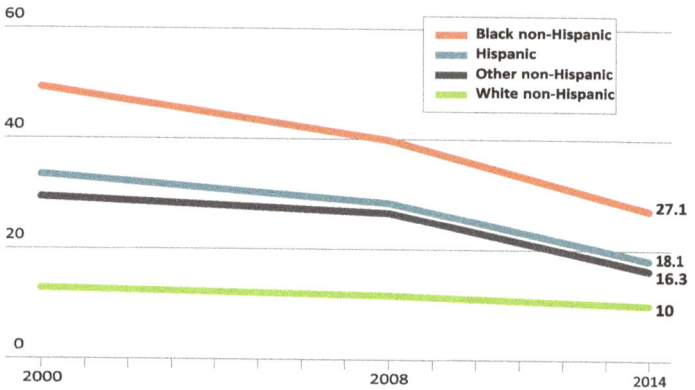

gu.tt/Abortion2014   ©2017

https://www.guttmacher.org/infographic/2017/abortion-rates-race-and-ethnicity

Leading Causes of Death for African Americans In the United States

Heart Disease	Drug Induced	Cancer	Diabetes
90,507	19,212	70,036	18,968
COVID	Homicide	Accidents	**ABORTIONS**
55,994	14,313	33,830	**262,911**

APPENDIX D – Major Religious Groups' Positions on Abortion according to Pew Research Center

Major religious groups' positions on abortion

Opposes abortion rights, with few or no exceptions	Supports abortion rights, with some limits	Supports abortion rights, with few or no limits	No clear position
• African Methodist Episcopal Church	• Episcopal Church	• Conservative Judaism	• Islam
• Assemblies of God	• Evangelical Lutheran Church in America	• Presbyterian Church (U.S.A.)	• Buddhism
• Roman Catholic Church	• United Methodist Church	• Reform Judaism	• National Baptist Convention
• Church of Jesus Christ of Latter-day Saints		• Unitarian Universalist	• Orthodox Judaism
• Hinduism		• United Church of Christ	
• Lutheran Church-Missouri Synod			
• Southern Baptist Convention			

Source: Pew Research Center review of outside literature

PEW RESEARCH CENTER

64

NOTES

_____

_____

_____

_____

_____

_____

_____

_____

_____

_____

_____

_____

_____

_____

_____

_____

_____

_____

_____

_____

_____

_____

_____

_____

Rev. Barbara J. Crawford, Ed. D., M. Div.

Dr. Barbara J. Conwell Crawford is a retired pastor and educator living in Goodlettsville, TN. She credits her favorite scripture, Romans 8:28, as inspiration for her life's work because she *truly* loves the Lord, believes she has been called according to *His* purpose and that all things *always* work together for the good!

Dr. Crawford served as Pastor of St. Luke African Methodist Episcopal (AME) Church, Gallatin, Tennessee, for five years prior to her retirement October 2023. Previously, the Nashville native served as pastor of St. Luke AME Church in Nashville, Tennessee, and St. Paul AME Church in Woodburn, Kentucky. An ordained Elder in the African Methodist Episcopal Church since 1996, Dr. Crawford faithfully served as Assistant Pastor of Payne Chapel AME Church, Nashville, for more than 20 years under the pastorate of Rev. Sidney F. Bryant. She now serves as an Associate Minister of Payne Chapel.

Dr. Crawford retired from the Metropolitan Nashville Public School System in 2007. During her 37 years with Metro Schools, she served as a teacher, reading specialist, and principal. She began her teaching career as one of the first African-American teachers assigned to a previously all-White school. Under her leadership as principal of Wharton Middle School, Wharton Arts Magnet (relocated and renamed Creswell Arts Magnet), Nashville's first and only middle school arts magnet program, was established.

A life-long learner, Dr. Crawford received a Bachelor of Science degree in Elementary Education from Tennessee (A&I) State University (1969), a Master's degree in Reading from Middle Tennessee State University (1976), a +30 Endorsement in Administration and Supervision from Tennessee State University (1986), and a Doctor of Education degree from Peabody College of Vanderbilt University (1991). She received a Master of Divinity degree from Vanderbilt University in 2014.

Dr. Crawford has been recognized for her service to children, the church, and the community. Her honors include: National Council of Christians and Jews Brotherhood-Sisterhood Educator of the Year Award, HCA Teacher Award, Frist Principal Award, and UPN Nashville Principal of the Month. In 2017 she was recognized for having completed the Goodlettsville Leadership Academy. Her first book, *But...You Don't Know My Story – Women Who Experienced Abortion Share Their Stories*, was published in 2024. Dr. Crawford is a member of Delta Sigma Theta Sorority, Inc.

An itinerant elder serving in the AME Tennessee Conference, Dr. Crawford was recognized in 2018 by the Conference's Lay Organization as a "Pastor of the Year." She has served as a member of the Tennessee Conference Board of Examiners, chair of the Conference Christian Education Committee, and Secretary and past President of the Gallatin United Ministerial Alliance.

Dr. Crawford and her husband, James, celebrated their 52th wedding anniversary June 9, 2025. They are the proud parents of two sons, Rev. Marlan E. Crawford and Michael A. Crawford, Sr.; daughter-in-love, Sarita; and three grown grandchildren, Michael Jr., Jordan Jeanee, and Mason.